How to Lose Weight the Healthy Way

The 10 Health Habits you Need to Develop

by Tarryn Thompson

Magic Press

Orlando, FL 32703

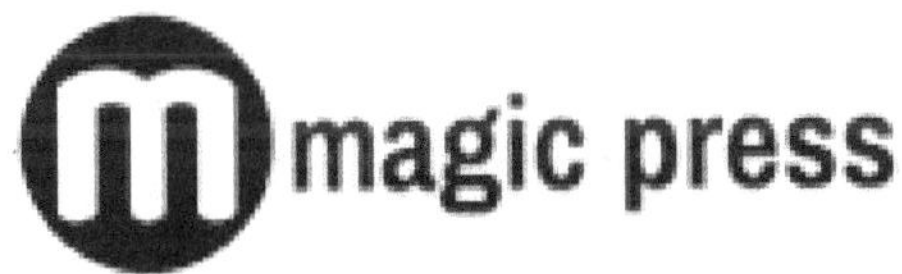

Tarryn Thompson
Generation Health Ltd
www.GenerationHealth.co.nz

"I felt so supported the whole way through"

I loved that I could reach out to Tarryn during the week as well. There were so many tools I had access to that helped me. I have so much more energy and I am sleeping so much better.

Before doing Tarryn's program I had been to Weight Watchers, Sure Slim and all those other things. The thing that was such a big draw card to Tarryn's program was the hormone approach. In the past the focus has always been about getting through a 12 week program or getting through a challenge and then once its all over I can go out and have a drink. It was always about losing the weight but never about my habits and so it made it about rewards instead of growth. I'm handling stress better, handling my relationships better. I don't sweat the small stuff like I did before. I am a whole different person now thanks to Tarryn's program and her support.

I've still got a way to go to reach my ideal but I feel equipped with the necessary skills and I'm still connected to Tarryn's support program to help me the rest of the way.

- Emma Fowler, wife, mother and manager of a child care facility.

"The weight loss and centimetres lost were a bonus"

Before starting Tarryn's program I had all sorts of gut issues. I felt depressed about my IBS and candida. It was taking over my life. Now I feel so much better. I know what to do to manage it and its totally changed the way I think about food.

I really loved how available Tarryn was for support. The program helped me understand more about my body and my condition. Plus it helped me with quite a few old beliefs I was carrying around about nutrition. I totally recommend it.

- Pippa McLeod, wife and mother of 3

"I lost 8cm from my hips. Thats never happened before"
Before starting Tarryn's program I felt like I had hit a rut and nothing was working. I felt really unmotivated because in the past I'd tried a lot of things and it hadn't worked. But this felt different.
I'm the sort of person that loves to understand everything before I follow it.
I absolutely loved that Tarryn's program taught me the 'why' behind everything. I've seen a dietician and gone to Jenny Craig before and never had the same kind of understanding behind it.
The program made a lot of sense and the principles behind it made me see that it's not all about losing weight but also about creating the habits necessary for a healthy lifestyle.

- Nicky Mayson, wife and mother of 2

"It's the best investment I have EVER made"
Before starting Tarryn's program I was overweight, I hated not being able to fit into any clothes and I exercised a lot but never seemed to lose any weight.
I used to wake up in the morning with a dull headache and really lethargic. I was also thinking about getting older and not wanting to be in a really unhealthy state especially when I got into my 50's.
So far I've lost 10kg and 20cm from my belly, I'm still losing and best of all it's given me the knowledge about my body and how to implement a lifestyle change.
It is the best investment I have EVER made and because of Tarryn's continued support I now have the confidence in myself to achieve any health goal I set my mind to.

- Sarah Greenway, wife, mother of 3 and office manager

Heres Whats Inside…

Introduction

Thank you for receiving my book. I especially want to commend you for taking the time to up-skill yourself and increase your knowledge about health, nutrition and your body.

If, like me, you have been working on this area of your life for your whole life, then I want to virtually hi-five you for trusting that there is value for you here.

My name is Tarryn Thompson; I'm a health coach and hormone specialist.

In this book I'm going to share with you 10 health habits that once developed can set you free from the world of yo-yo dieting so that you can finally start living in the body you desire.

These 10 health habits form the basis of education covered in my signature online coaching program.

Once implemented, they can create for you a lifestyle that has the side effect of permanent fat loss, boundless energy, and most importantly – finally feeling free from the world of yo-yo dieting.

I get to speak with a lot of people and hear their concerns and see the approaches they've taken in the past to address their weight. What I see most people doing is going against their body and not working with it to allow it to do these things.

Over the last 7 years I've specialised in educating people about how fat is burned, how to address specific hormonal weaknesses and coaching them to develop a winning weight loss mindset.

My personal journey has been a big one. To date, I've shed just over 30 kilos. But that's not where my story ended. Even though I'd reached my goal weight I still hated the way my body looked.

My problem areas had always been my hips, bum and thighs and it was incredibly frustrating. I was lean and strong and the fittest I had ever been, but I had a problem with cellulite and I just couldn't shift it.

This internal battle resulted in me having a consultation with a surgeon about liposuction.

Well thankfully I didn't go through with the surgery.

I used this challenge to lead me to discover an area of health that I'd completely overlooked. It's an area that once addressed, allowed my body to let go of the fat in my problem areas.

I discovered there were other hormone imbalances I needed to correct and my body needed an even more specific environment for it to release fat from my lower half.

Once I incorporated this into my own regime I was able to lose the fat from my legs WITHOUT surgery, and finally get into my bikini with confidence. ;-)

I want you to know that I get your frustration …

I've been at rock bottom many times, I was convinced surgery was my only solution.

I'm guessing you've probably tried many different programs and plans, perhaps even seen health professionals. If you're anything like me you probably can take the amount of money you've spent on your health and have put down a deposit on a house.
Here's an inconvenient truth I've discovered in my life: You cannot have success without failure, or breakthroughs without challenges and if you continue to resist against challenges in this area it will always be difficult.

If you continue to choose ease over difficulty, and support over challenge it becomes a habitual way of thinking and very difficult to break free of.

Challenges will continue to find you until you choose to find the lesson your failures are trying to show you.

When you acknowledge and be truly grateful for both challenge and failure, then you'll be able to interrupt that cycle of behaviour and push through to solve your problem.

Without challenge you cannot grow and every one of your past attempts to lose weight has brought you to this point right now.

Perhaps your weight loss challenges are showing you that lesson.

If you're feeling challenged in this area of your life, know that you're right where you need to be and a breakthrough is just around the corner.

The question is: will you embrace the challenge and push through?

I hope so, because the ability to bounce back after a failure is one of the most important character traits anyone can possess in life.

To Your Success

Tarryn

Change Your Focus, Change Your Results

I'd like to suggest to you a different approach to weight loss. An approach that has you winning in the long term.

That is a habit based approach. It's your habits that determine your results. It's not what you do one time or for 7 days or 12 weeks. It's what you do consistently over a long enough period of time that gets you to your goal.

If you focus solely on your results then when you step on the scale and you're not happy with what you see it doesn't leave you feeling very good.

If you don't feel good then you're unlikely to make the necessary decisions over a long enough period of time for them to become habits.

When you focus on creating the right health habits you can always see progress no matter what the results might show.

The truth is, your results are a reflection of your habits so if you can change them, then no matter how big your goal is you can reach it.

I hope by the time you finish reading this book, you can acknowledge that there is a way for you to reach your ideal body. And a habit based approach is that way. Ask yourself....have the other approaches you've tried in the past addressed weight loss in this way? My guess is ... probably not.

What you're about to discover are the 10 Health Habits that once developed will pay you back with lasting weight loss and freedom from the world of yo-yo dieting.

So here they are ...

HABIT #1
I eat within 30 minutes of waking up, and I do not eat within 2 hours of going to bed

The first habit has nothing to do with what you eat but when you eat. It's based on a principle called 'book ending your day' and it suggests that, although we can be limited by what we can control during the day, we can be totally in control on how we start and finish it.

I am well aware that preparing breakfast in the morning can be a pain and sometimes after a long day at work, making dinner is the last thing you want to do. But mastering this habit helps to keep blood sugars stable through the day and clears sugar from your blood at night.

If you eat within 30 minutes of waking (without spiking your blood sugar) you're ability to make better decisions about the next meal becomes easier.

If you don't learn to stabilise your blood sugars, mid morning cravings are inevitable. By the afternoon your blood sugars are on the floor leaving you tired and exhausted. Your desire to snack on sweet or nutrient empty foods to keep yourself going will be at an all time high. As a result your moods can become like a roller coaster – up and down, just like your energy. And you'll probably feel a strong urge for caffeine just to make it through the day.

Insulin triggered in excess at night can cancel out all your fat burning efforts from throughout the day.

If your last meal for the day is 2 hours before bed it means digestion would have finished by the time you reach that deep restorative sleep, and the majority, if not all of your insulin cleared from your blood.

This means that while you sleep you'll be capitalising on all of your fat burning efforts from earlier in the day.

I want you to remember this. Fat will not burn in the presence of too much insulin, and seeing as you do most of your fat burning while you sleep, if you have excessive insulin in your blood your body cannot access its fat stores for healing and repair.

Stabilising your blood sugars is super important. Almost all of your hormone imbalances will show improvement if you're able to do so.

If insulin is cleared from the blood during the night you'll wake up with more energy, you'll feel like the brain cloud has lifted and your thoughts are clearer. Cortisol levels decrease and your adrenal glands can begin to strengthen. Many women notice their libido start to return and of course your vitality and your moods stabilise.

The best way I've found to start the day is with a breakfast smoothie. Its quick and easy but it's got to be balanced. What you eat in the morning should not spike your blood sugar.

You can make your own or use a premixed shake powder. There are certain guidelines I suggest you follow when making your own smoothie which I've outlined in my **How To Make Your Own Smoothie Guide.** You can find that in the resources section at the end of the book.

If you need a convenient option, premixed shakes may be a great strategy for you. A whole food smoothie is better but if it means you're getting something in your system that tastes great, is packed with nutrients and doesn't spike your blood sugar then seriously, it's ok.

I recommend the meal replacement shakes from Usana Health Sciences. They've got a Low GI rating of just 25 and all 3 flavours taste delicious.
You can **buy USANA Foods from my online store.** The link is in the resources section.

If you have more time in the morning then any egg based breakfast is a great start. It's low carb, medium protein and high fat. It won't spike your blood sugar and it'll keep you feeling fuller for longer.

Here's one of my favourites:
Vegetable Omelette with Spinach & Avocado Spread. The recipe is in the resources section.

You can literally play around with any combination of eggs, additional good fat sources and low glycemic vegetables.

If you're exercising later in the evening or you work a night shift I suggest making your last meal of the day an easily digestible one. Especially the protein portion of your meal. Some easy digestible proteins are eggs, sashimi, tahini, hummus, legumes and pulses. If this is a late post exercise meal the good news is insulin clearing is exceptionally efficient at this time.

Now I get asked about intermittent fasting a lot which kind of flies in the face of this habit. The truth is intermittent fasting is a great weight loss strategy. I do it and I teach it to my intermediate and advanced students.

But it is just that. An intermediate and advanced strategy. I recommend it once you are practiced at the basics of nutrition. I don't believe fasting is a sustainable strategy for most people most of the time. So I fall back on the habit of eating within 30mins of waking when I am not fasting.

KEY LEARNINGS

- We may not be able to control what happens during the day but we can control how it starts and finishes.
- If you don't learn to stabilise your blood sugars, mid morning cravings are inevitable.
- Insulin triggered at night can cancel out all your fat burning efforts from throughout the day.
- If insulin is cleared from the blood during the night you'll wake up with more energy
- Start your day with a breakfast smoothie

HABIT #2
I eat every 3 hours. If I'm hungry before then I'll eat and adjust my time accordingly

This second health habit deals with 3 separate things: **Meal preparation, meal frequency and mindfulness around eating.**

When you are mindful and consider what your body is trying to tell you it gives you an opportunity to respond accordingly.

The main cue you'll experience is hunger. If you're hungry too soon between meals it often means 1 of 2 things: What you ate in your previous meal needs to be adjusted to satiate you longer. Or your metabolism is starting to speed up.

Other cues you can experience are cravings for carbs or sugar, tiredness or fatigue and bloating.

To implement this habit, start by keeping a food journal for at least 2-3 days. Preferably 2 work days and 1 non-work day. While food journaling you'll be able to make the connection between hunger cravings and what and when you eat.

You'll find most of your problems come from missing a snack, going too long without eating, overeating and not eating enough especially post exercise.

Next, make a meal plan. There are basically 3 meal plan structures I recommend.

Menu A - Using meal replacement shakes and snack bars (Highly recommended to jumpstart 1-3 weeks but not recommended long term)

Menu B - Using a combination of meal replacement shakes and snack bars with meals and snacks you make yourself. (Recommended as you transition to Menu C)

Menu C - Making all meals and snacks yourself. (This is the ultimate goal but not always a reality for some people. A combination of Menu B and C works for most)

Once you've chosen a Menu Structure the next thing to do is **Meal Scheduling.**

(Menu structures and meal schedule found in the resources section)

Start by book ending your day and schedule your first meal within 30 minutes of waking and your last meal 2 hours before bed. Then schedule the rest of your meals and snacks with the hours left in between. Just do your best with this, especially if you have dedicated break times at work or any other variables that dictates when you can or can't eat. As long as your meals and snacks are roughly 3 hours apart that's good enough to begin with.

As you implement your plan, notice your body's cues and adjust meals and eating times accordingly.

If you don't get into the habit of eating mindfully and allocating time to prepare your meals then many people find their mind is constantly on food. Wondering what to eat next is a common time waster. Reflect on your previous week and ask yourself how much of the time your mind is on food and how you feel as a result?

How much time are you contemplating what you should eat, when you should eat, how much you should eat? When I get stuck in this cycle of thinking it leads me to wish I had more confidence, more willpower, discipline and motivation.

By being prepared, you create mind-space for other important things in life. You might notice your thoughts become others focused, maybe even about how you can contribute more. Perhaps you begin showing patience, compassion and understanding with others who are going through their own struggles.

These emotions all require energy and it's really difficult to consider others when you are feeling challenged and struggling yourself.

You may even start to entertain thoughts of trying new things and find yourself having more experiences with your new found confidence - as opposed to being consumed by your body and all things about it that hold you back.

When we take a focused period of time to prepare how we will nourish our body for the day ahead, when we take a pause....we begin the process of creating a healthy relationship with food and a greater appreciation for our body as we listen and respond to the cues it's sending us.

Amazingly, when you give your body what it wants, in turn it will give you what you want.

There's one variable to be aware of with this habit. If you have a hormone imbalance related to the liver or thyroid, then the speed of your metabolism will be slower. You will need to make sure your main meal times are at least 5 hours apart with no excessive snacking.

If you're unsure what hormonal imbalance may be affecting your weight loss success then Click here to **take our body type quiz** and find out your primary body type. (quiz link in the resources section)

KEY LEARNINGS

- Be mindful and consider what your body is trying to tell you.
- Start by keeping a food journal for at least 2-3 days
- Choose a meal plan structure and schedule your meal times.
- Implement your plan, notice your body's cues and adjust meals and eating times accordingly.
- Watch out for missed snacks, going too long without eating, overeating and not eating enough after exercise.

BONUS - Meal Preparation Tips

- Buy all your food for the whole week and prepare 3 days in advance to save time.
- The quantity of food to prepare will differ from person to person so use hunger cues as your guide. It may take a few weeks to get your quantities and frequency on point. And be prepared because it will change again and you'll need to make adjustments.
- These preparation tips will help you save time, be more efficient, and increase your chances of sticking to your plan.

Breakfast Prep

- Make it easy on yourself and have a smoothie in the morning. Refer to Habit #1 for balanced smoothie making guidelines or use a premixed shake
- If you're not making smoothies for breakfast then try this omelette prep: Make enough for 3 omelettes at one time.
- STEP 1: Prepare the veggies. I love onion, mushroom, capsicum and spinach so just sauté them with some butter. This will go inside the omelette so set this aside once it's done.
- STEP 2: Depending on your body type use 2-3 whole eggs per omelette and cook on low heat. Season the egg with salt and pepper to taste. If you have a large enough pan make all 3 omelettes at once.

- STEP 3: Add the vegetables to the inside. Add cheese if you'd like.
- STEP 4: Fold over the omelette as soon as the eggs start to brown.
- STEP 5: Divide into 3 even amounts and put into containers. Refrigerate, and when you're ready, warm them on the stove.
- Depending on how long they kept you going will determine how much cheese and whether you should continue to use both cheese and butter.
- With portion sizes of fats such as cheese and butter, use your thumb as a guide.
- Generally I recommend 1-3 serves of fat per main meal.

Lunch Prep
- STEP 1: Start with some frozen or fresh fish fillets, sautéd in some butter and sprinkled with a few herbs and spices such as dill, fennel, garlic, pepper. The basic serving size is 1-1.5 palms sizes of fish your body type.
- Make sure the fish is not overdone - remember you will be re-heating the fish and you don't want it to go rubbery.
- Divide the fish into 3 containers, then put them in the fridge.
- STEP 2: Make a quick coleslaw from shredded cabbage and carrot, diced red onion and coriander. You can also use a bag of pre-mixed coleslaw mix to save time.
- STEP 3: If you use the packet dressing make sure it contains no sugar or MSG. To make your own dressing: combine whole egg mayonnaise, lemon juice and white vinegar.
- STEP 4: When you're ready to eat, add 1 cup of coleslaw to a container, pour 3 teaspoons of dressings on top, shake, reheat your fish fillet and you're done.
- Depending on your hunger, you may want to add some hummus on the side. You can make your own using chickpeas and tahini or buy pre-made at the supermarket. About 2 tablespoons of hummus is enough.
- In this instance it's mayonnaise and tahini that is the fat portion of the meal and the oil if that's what you cooked the fish in.

Snack Prep
- Many people will get hungry if they don't have enough healthy fats in their diet.
- Try a combination of peanut butter (no added sugar) mixed with tahini butter.
- Tahini butter is made from sesame seeds and can be found at any supermarket usually in the organic section.
- Adding tahini butter to your meals will lower the glycemic effect even further because it's moderate in protein and high in good fats. The lower the glycemic effect of a meal, the longer you'll feel satisfied from your meal.
- Mix the 2 butters together 50/50.
- Try the peanut/sesame butter mix with carrot, celery or cucumber sticks.

Dinner Prep
- STEP 1: Start by cutting up some vegetables. I like capsicum, carrot, cucumber, mushrooms and red onion.
- STEP 2: Divide the cut vegetables into 3 containers. Aim to have at least 2 cups of cut vegetables per container.
- STEP 3: Add 2-4 cups of a leafy green salad to each container of cut vegetables. Do not add dressing until you're ready to consume.
- You may want to add some sunflower seeds (preferably raw) and feta cheese to up the fat content. You can use either your thumb to portion out the fat or a TBS. For example 1 TBS of seeds and 1 thumbed portion of feta.
- STEP 4: Prepare enough cooked protein for 3 days
- STEP 5: Add the cooked protein to your prepared salad each day
- STEP 6: Add any no-sugar dressing and enjoy

HABIT #3
I eat according to my goals. Low Glycemic Load (GL) to lose weight, and Medium GL to maintain

Hands down this health habit is the most important health habit to create. It helps you manage your carbohydrate intake. It's so important because carbs spike your blood sugar and trigger the most amount of fat storing hormones.

When you make fat storing hormones there's no way your body will choose to burn fat.

You have many opportunities to eat therefore you have many opportunities to spike your blood sugar. The best tool I have found to manage carb intake is the Glycemic Load. The Glycemic Load or GL refers to the quantity of carbohydrates consumed at one time. You may have heard of the Glycemic Index before, if you haven't it is referring to the speed at which carbohydrates convert to blood glucose.

While both are important, I place a greater focus on the Glycemic Load because the Glycemic Index does not take into account the quantity of carbs consumed.

I really struggled with carbs because they were such a staple part of my up bringing, so at the beginning I did find it a challenge to reduce those portions. But as I did, I discovered the Glycemic Load of my meals were a real trigger for cravings and overeating.

Having this tool encouraged me to start being mindful of the carbohydrate portion of my meals and snacks and I'm confident it can do the same for you too. At first it can seem like a lot of work, checking charts and adding up the GL for your meals, but the more you do it the more you'll start to notice patterns. Soon you will see that it's not really difficult at all, it was just unfamiliar.

I've done all the heavy lifting for you by creating the **Carbohydrate Cheat Sheet.** Download it from the resources section, print it and stick it to your fridge. Then each time you prepare a meal reference it until you get your head around this habit.

You'll notice the main culprits leading to excessive carb intake are grains and starches. It's easy to manipulate the serving size of these carbs and just replace them with extra lower GL vegetables which can be eaten in abundance.

If your goal is to lose weight then aim to keep the GL of all meals and snacks under 10GL.

To maintain your weight you have a little more flexibility with Glycemic Load. You can fluctuate your meals between 0-10 and 11-17. These numbers will make sense when you download the cheat sheet. Remember, the GL is the sum total of the carbohydrate component of your meal.

If you need help identifying what foods are carbs, I've laid it out very simply for you in the **Carbohydrate Cheat Sheet** along with the portions sizes and GL for each.

NOTE: The glycemic load targets I've given refer to the sum of each meal or snack, not your whole day.

Now if you're not too jazzed about the idea of checking charts and adding up the GL of all meals and snacks then here are a few challenges you may face.

A world of low energy and lethargy. Spending each day trying to resist cravings and constantly dealing with the guilt of caving in.

Here's a taste of what's ahead if you do: Imagine this. You wake up naturally, perhaps even before your alarm clock. You get out of bed calmly, you're brain fog has lifted, and while you're aware of all the things you need to do, it does not bring any sense of overwhelm.

As you observe yourself in the mirror you're sure you look skinnier. You don't even need to weigh yourself because you know you've lost weight.. But maybe you do anyway because you're not yet out of that habit.

Your clothes are feeling noticeably looser. You prepare your breakfast smoothie and grab the lunch you prepared the the night before. Your close friends and colleagues are noticing the changes and dish out a few complements.

You may notice your energy is stable throughout the day and you're not craving like you used to.
You're workmate hands around some leftover birthday cake, you may not even feel like it and pass up the offer. You're the invited out for a coffee for afternoon break and you choose the coffee because you enjoy it not because you need it. Big difference.

You arrive home and you're feeling good. You prepared a big salad yesterday and all you need to do is piece the roast chicken you bought on your way home and dinner is done. You sit down and relax and continue reading my book.

Sound good?

Great!

Start by downloading the **Carbohydrate Cheat Sheet** from the resources section, and stick it to your fridge.

KEY LEARNINGS

- You must learn to manage your carbohydrate intake by learning the Glycemic Load of your meals.
- To lose weight keep the total GL of each meal and snack under 10.
- The main culprits leading to excessive carb intake are grains and starches.
- Manipulate the serving size of these carbs and replace them with lower GL vegetables.

HABIT #4
I eat enough protein with my meals

The fourth habit to develop is a real game changer because protein helps you feel fuller for longer. It takes longer for your body to digest protein so when consumed with carbs it slows down the rate of digestion, therefore you'll get through the day feeling satisfied when getting enough protein.

This is important because it creates a low insulin environment – and remember fat will not burn in the presence of insulin.

Protein might just become your favourite macronutrient because when you are eating the correct proportion, protein will also trigger fat burning hormones.

But wait there's more, when fat burning hormones are elevated, fat storage hormones are suppressed.

Unfortunately for most people, the average amount of protein consumed per day is just 30 grams. It's way too low and it often comes in one main meal. Usually in the evening. You should be consuming between 50 - 75 grams per day. There are some variables but this is an average recommendation.

If you don't get enough protein with your meals and snacks, life can get pretty tough. Typical breakfast options are usually low in protein. Breakfast smoothies are popular but they usually consist of too much fruit.

By morning break, most people are reaching for something to bring energy up again. Biscuits, bread, crackers, muffins, doughnuts, waffles and scones are usually what goes down.

Lunchtime is generally the first time of day to have a proper meal with a good source of protein but because nothing was pre prepared, grabbing something "on the run" has become a common habit for city dwellers. In fact sushi seems to tick the boxes as being the "healthiest" most "convenient" option to choose.

Then afternoon 3:30itis kicks in. It's such an internal battle to make a good food decision at this point. Blood sugar levels are on the floor and caffeine can be the only perceived thing that will get someone through the day.

If you can relate to this day, it's because blood sugars have been all over the place and a big part of it is because we have not eaten enough protein.

Dinner is often the time protein makes her grand entrance. But unfortunately as the curtains open and she steps out on stage, the audience is asleep because it's been such a long day. We hit the sack with a 200 gram steak to digest and we wonder why feel sluggish in the morning.

I am literally feeling exhausted just writing about this exhausting day.

If you hit the mark with protein intake, your day will look drastically different. But be careful not to over consume protein either. An over consumption of this macronutrient can lead to excessive insulin production so it's important to get the balance right.

Protein intake does vary from person to person. Your level of activity and whether you're male or female are the usual variables but also take into account your body type.

If you are storing fat around your midsection predominantly, or if you are storing fat around your hips, buttocks and thighs your intake should be between 50-75 grams of protein per day.

For instance, if you consumed 100 grams of weighted chicken, that would be the equivalent of 21 grams of protein contributing to approximately ⅓ of your daily intake.

If you have a 'pot belly' or a fatty roll under the bust, or, if you don't really store fat in any one particular place but you store it globally - your daily protein intake should be between 50 and 75 grams but no more than 25 - 35 grams from animal protein. The rest must come from vegetarian or easily digestible sources like legumes, pulses, hummus, fish especially sashimi, eggs, tahini butter, nuts and seeds.

The main challenge you'll face in implementing this habit is being prepared with your protein sources. Most proteins require preparation and cooking time but once you do you can store 2-3 days worth in the refrigerator. A lot of the time I cheat and buy a cooked free range chicken on my way home. It usually covers us for dinner and lunch the next day.

To stay extra organised, keep your pantry stocked up with tins of tuna, salmon, chicken, black beans, kidney beans, lentils and your freezer stocked with fish portions, lean beef or lamb patties.

Here are some **Desirable Protein Sources** I use and recommend. Beans, Lentils, Eggs (free range), Gurnard, Tarakihi, Mackerel, Salmon, Sardines, Snapper, Blue Cod, Lamb, Lean beef cuts (fillet, sirloin, rump), Turkey, Venison, Chicken (free range).

KEY LEARNINGS

- Protein helps you feel fuller for longer.
- When eaten in the correct proportion, protein can trigger fat burning hormones.
- Be careful not to over consume protein either or it can stimulate fat storing hormones
- Consume between 50 - 75 grams per day.
- Take into account your body type.
- Prepare your protein source in advance and stay stocked up with convenient protein options.

HABIT #5
I eat good fats with my meals and snacks, especially the omega 3's

The fifth habit to develop is also a real game changer because good fats also help you feel fuller longer. When consumed with carbs and protein they further slow down your rate of digestion, therefore you'll get through the day feeling even more satisfied.

Fats are actually hormonally neutral, meaning they don't stimulate fat burning or fat making hormones unless they're consumed with a high glycemic meal.

There is actually another underlying principle around this habit. It has to do with keeping inflammation low in your body. The omega 3 fats are anti-inflammatory which reduces cortisol.
This is important because less cortisol means less fat storing hormone in your body.

To get these anti-inflammatory benefits you must correct the ratio of omega 3 fats to omega 6 fats in your diet. Due to; 1) the amount of cooking we do using vegetable oils, and 2) the reduction in fish consumption, our ratio of 6's to 3's are very disproportioned. Omega 6's are just more readily available. Like almonds, olive oil, peanut butter and avocado.

To get the benefits from good fats, we need to have our ratios of 6's : 3's be closer to a 5:1 or even better still a 3:1 ratio.

A better ratio of 6's to 3's means the membranes of our cells remain supple. This helps with nutrients being absorbed into your cells. It also greatly improves your muscle cell's ability to receive sugar which very simply means less sugar to be up-taken into your fat cells. A better ratio of omega 6's to 3's also means better manufacturing of sex hormones.

This can make the difference between feeling sexy and happy or depressed and angry.

Other subtle side effects of low good fat intake can also manifest themselves as poor skin, tired eyes, skin conditions like eczema, sore joints and brain fog just to name a few.

Over time, low good fat intake can lead to hormonal acne, high LDL (bad) cholesterol and low HDL (good) cholesterol, low sex drive and libido, fertility problems, compromised gut health, behavioural conditions especially with children, and neurological conditions as well.

The best way to address this habit is to first become aware of the different fats. Omega 6's, omega 3's and saturated fats.

Saturated fats are not the evil fats they're been marketed to be. There are tremendous health benefits to coconut products and grass fed butter.

Start by downloading **The Good Fats Cheat Sheet** print it out and stick it on your fridge. You'll find it super helpful to start correcting your Omega 6:3 ratio.

The next thing to do is stop using vegetable oils for high-heat cooking and replace it with a saturated fat like coconut oil or butter. Saturated fats are much more stable at high temperatures. Only use vegetable oils for dressings or for low-heat cooking with the exception of extra virgin olive oil which is ok at moderate heat.

Then add a practitioner grade fish oil supplement to your daily supplement regime. It's simply the most convenient way to bring your ratio of omega 6's to 3's back into line on a consistent basis. I recommend a minimum of 2 x 1 gram capsules (which is equivalent to eating 2x100gm servings of salmon per day).

The high quality fish oil supplement I use and recommend to my clients is from Usana Health Sciences. They call it **BiOmega™**

You can **buy BiOmega™ from my online store here.** (Link in the resources section)

BiOmega is produced from sustainably raised, cold-water, deep-sea sardines. It's purified to be free of contaminants so you don't have to worry about mercury poisoning.

The balance of DHA and EPA is more than many competitors and personally, I like the fact that BiOmega is also fortified with vitamin D and it has an added lemon flavouring, so there is no fishy breath for me.

If you master this habit then you can experience what often gets referred to as "the glow". Clear skin, shiny hair, strong nails, eyes bright. Hormones will start to become more balanced and you may also notice your libido start to return.

If you're an estrogen body type like me then you really need to double your fish oil intake to 4 grams per day. It's what I take. Trust me, your skin and your ass will love you for it.

Estrogen and Adrenal body types need a total of 5 - 7 servings of fats spread out over the day. 1 serving is equivalent to the size of your thumb or 1 TBSP. In the instance of measuring hard fat sources like avocado, nuts, and cheeses, use the thumb measurement. In the instance of measuring seeds, oils, or dressings like mayonnaise, the TBSP measurement would be the best option.

Liver and Thyroid body types need slightly lower levels of dietary good fats. 3-5 servings of fats spread out over the day. If you have no problems with bowel movements or digestion you could add an extra 2 servings with snacks or your main meals.

If you're unsure what hormonal imbalance may be affecting your weight loss success then Click here to **take the body type quiz** and find out your primary body type. (Quiz link in the resources section)

KEY LEARNINGS

- Good fats help you feel fuller longer.
- Good fats don't stimulate fat burning or fat making hormones unless they're consumed with a high glycemic meal.
- Good fats help reduce inflammation.
- Improve the ratio of omega 3 fats to omega 6 fats in your diet.
- Eat the right amount of dietary fat for your body type.
- Take a practitioner grade fish oil supplement at least 2 times per day.

HABIT #6
I get at least 35 grams of fibre per day

Getting enough fibre in your diet is one of the things that you'll wish you knew about sooner, and **when you experience the benefits of fibre you'll never want to go without it.**

Fibre is a carbohydrate, however it is indigestible, which means the body doesn't absorb it so it does not convert to sugar into your bloodstream like other carbohydrates. In fact, fibre does one better. When consumed with other carbs, fibre will act like a buffer and slow the whole process of digestion down.

Fibre also creates bulk to the stool. A bulky stool stimulates muscle contractions to easily move waste through the large intestine naturally and effortlessly.

And finally, **one fact that might just change your life. Fibre is the food that feeds the good bacteria that live in your gut.**

How is this life changing you ask? Well let me explain.

Starting from about ½ way through your digestive process, food is broken down into small enough particle sizes by the stomach before moving through to the small intestines. Here, the partly digested food moves through the intestines being further processed by the bacteria that live there. The bacteria's job is to break down the food particles into their smallest sizes we call your micronutrients. These are the vitamin and mineral components of your food.

But wait a minute … there's not enough good bacteria … because they have been starved to death as a result of not getting enough fibre in your diet. Fibre is the food for the good bacteria.

There's a mutual relationship you have with your good bacteria, they break down your food so you can absorb it and benefit from the nutrition. You eat fibre giving them their food so that they can survive and continue to do their job.

If you have not been coming to the party with your side of the deal then you can severely inhibit your body's ability to uptake the vitamins and minerals that your body needs to perform basic functions.

You could also experience break fog, low immunity and constantly being unwell. Unbalanced sex hormones, stress, gut problems such as irritable bowel syndrome and leaky gut.

Diverticulitis is also common. Problems with elimination such as constipation, bloating and discomfort. Also a stressed liver because fat soluble waste is not able to be efficiently excreted from the bowels.

As a result of low fibre intake your body can have a lot of trouble letting go of fat when it's stressed out because of the problems happening with your digestive system. This stress creates more opportunity for fat storage hormones to be produced.

If you become a master of this health habit, I said your life will change. And I meant it.

A flat stomach all day long because waste is efficiently clearing, going for number 2's in about the same time it takes you to urinate (no joke! – it will be that efficient when your bowels are in working order, hardly any wipes necessary so you'll also save money on toilet paper, hehe).

An improved immune system so when you do get sick it won't completely take you out. Colds and flus become less and less frequent until you hardly get sick at all. You're able to last longer in between meals as a result of stable blood sugars. You'll have more energy because you are actually able to absorb the nutrients from your food. Hormones start to balance because your organs and glands are able to receive the vitamins and minerals from your food so they can do their job.

The best way to address this habit is to know your starting point. You'll be surprised how low fibre intake is, in most people's diets. Typically 10-12 grams is where most of my one on one coaching clients are at when they first start working with me.

Keep a food journal of a typical day and then do a fibre count. It's easy to do, just download the **Fibre Cheat Sheet** to get started. (Link in the resources section)

Then begin adding more high fibre foods into your day. You'll see that pulses and legumes are your highest fibre foods. See where you can add a serving of these into your meals. Whole grains are your next best option but not at the expense of your overall GL. You'll need to make sure the serving size is kept in line with your goals.

Then the increase of vegetables (covered in the next habit) will contribute to you moving closer to the magic amount of 35 grams.

Now after all that you'll likely find yourself sitting around the 20-30 gram mark so a fibre supplement is what I recommend to bring you across the line. 35 grams is the minimum recommendation but if you want to take your life to a whole new level then I dare you to see what it's like at 50 grams per day. But take your time to get there.

The fibre supplement I use and recommend to my clients is from Usana Health Sciences. They call it **Fibergy™ Plus.**

You can **buy Fibergy™ Plus from my online store here.** (Link in the resources section)

If you have existing gut conditions, you really, really need to increase your fibre. Like your life depends on it. However you may not have enough enzymes just yet to be able to break the fibre down. So start with 20 grams and work up to 35 grams over 2-3 weeks. Then push to 50 grams when you feel ready.

Because of the overgrowth of bad bacteria people benefit from taking a course of probiotics to repopulate the good bacteria.

Especially if you've had your appendix removed. I had mine out when I was a teenager. I always wondered why my gut health was never amazing. Your appendix actually plays a key role in your gut and immune health.

Did you know your appendix is where your good bacteria go to hide when taking antibiotics?

Lastly, depending on the severity of your gut condition, you may need to double or triple the probiotic dose for 30 - 90 days. Definitely look around for other sources of probiotics as well, like kombucha, kefir and fermented vegetables.

The probiotic supplement I use and recommend to my clients is from Usana Health Sciences. They call it **USANA Probiotic.**

You can **buy USANA Probiotic from my online store here.** (Link in the resources section)

KEY LEARNINGS

- Fibre helps to slow down your digestive process, keeping you fuller for longer.
- It adds bulk to your stool helping you eliminate waste more effectively.
- Fibre is the food that feeds the good bacteria that live in your gut.
- Good bacteria break down your food so you can absorb it and benefit from the nutrition.
- Aim for at least 35 grams of fibre per day.

HABIT #7
I stay hydrated throughout the day

The seventh habit is probably not what you think it is. This habit is actually more about your vegetable intake than it is about drinking water. Drinking water is still important but it doesn't have to be X litres per day like you've been told before. Your daily water intake depends on the climate you're in, how much exercise you do, whether you're pregnant, etc, etc. Just drink water when you're thirsty.

So you might be wondering, what do vegetables have to do with hydration? And the answer is everything!

Has somebody ever told you your body is made up of 70% water? Well actually, that's not entirely accurate. You're made up of 70% electrolytes, comprised of key minerals like calcium, magnesium, sodium and potassium. And vegetables are your main sources of these minerals.

The balance of sodium / potassium is critical for better hydration. They basically go together like yin and yang. When potassium is low, sodium reins and it minimises the absorption of nutrients into the cell. Not to mention the stress this places on your kidneys. When you get adequate amounts of potassium, your cells are able to better absorb the water you drink.

The amount of potassium you need daily is around 5000mg. To get that you need to **consume a minimum of 7 serves of vegetables per day** (1 serve = 1 fist). If you're a larger person then aim for 8 servings and if you have a very high exercise output then 8-10 servings is your goal.

The best way to implement this habit is to focus on 2 - 3 serves of vegetables per main meal. In a breakfast smoothie you can easily blend 2 - 3 handfuls of spinach or kale in there so that gets you off to a great start.

Salads and soups are my other 2 strategies. Make a large batch every 2 - 3 days to save on time and use your GL Cheat Sheet to decide which vegetables are ok to use for your goals. I also really love purees. They're an easy way to consume vegetables quickly. Try this cauliflower and broccoli puree recipe: Boil 1 head of cauliflower and broccoli until tender. Then blend with 1/2 tsp of salt, 1 TBSP of butter and 100mls of coconut cream. Serves 4-6 depending on the size of your vegetables. Double the butter and coconut cream if you are serving 6.

The other important minerals you need for optimal hydration are calcium and magnesium. You will get them from vegetables for sure, but getting optimal levels of calcium and magnesium can be a challenge even with 7+ servings of vegetables.

The majority of our dietary calcium comes from dairy products. **Unfortunately the dairy form of calcium is not as well absorbed by the body and they're very acid-forming which can lead to weight gain, bone loss and loss of muscle tissue.**

Magnesium is even more scarce in our diets today and the scary thing is that not a single system in the body is able to function properly without magnesium. This is why it is important to eat plenty of magnesium-rich foods and supplements.

Magnesium supplementation delivers high enough doses to help keep stress hormones under control, reduce tension related headaches, alleviate depression and anxiety. It also supports our detoxification systems and energy production.

Magnesium also helps with the absorption of other nutrients such as calcium, copper, zinc, potassium and vitamin D as well. As a result it improves our immune system. It aids the digestive system, helps regulate blood sugar, heck, I could go on and on about magnesium.

The calcium and magnesium supplement I use and highly recommend comes from Usana Health Sciences. They call it **MagneCal D™** and provides balanced levels of calcium and magnesium, along with advanced levels of vitamin D in a truly bioavailable form.

You can **buy MagneCal D™ from my online store here.** (Link in the resources section)

Here are some of challenges you may experience if you don't develop this habit and stay hydrated:

- Fluid retention in your ankles and fingers.
- Puffy eyes.
- High blood pressure.
- Difficulty sleeping due to the amount of stress hormone that is being produced.
- As a result your adrenals are likely to be overworking which can leave you feeling anxious or with feelings of excessive stress.
- Your liver will be under pressure and will start to increase its production of cholesterol.
- Problems with cravings.
- Excessive urination, especially during the night.
- Water weight and an overall bloated look.

If you decide to develop this habit and stay hydrated you will notice more energy as your cells are actually electrically charged by potassium. Your muscles will be able to contract and relax easier with less cramping and restlessness.

Your skin will improve as the liver will be able to get more of the nutrients it needs. Your liver can also start to open up its detox pathways. Instead of being loaded and backlogged, the liver can start to prioritise the conversion of your fat into a form that you can excrete.

Here's another benefit to your liver getting what it needs. Cellulite reduction. This really plagued me for a long time. Cellulite is pockets of fluid formed around your fat and it usually exists in an environment of estrogen dominance. When your liver is getting the nutrients it needs and opens up its detox pathways, it can then prioritise excretion of estrogen instead of recirculating it back into your body.

KEY LEARNINGS

- The balance of sodium - potassium is critical for better hydration.
- Consume a minimum of 7 serves of vegetables per day for optimal levels of potassium.
- Eat plenty of magnesium-rich foods and supplements.
- Staying hydrated through optimal mineral intake helps to improve liver function and burn fat.

HABIT #8
I take a high potency, pharmaceutical grade multivitamin 2x a day

This habit is hands down **the easiest of all the habits to implement** and can potentially make the biggest impact to your health and weight loss efforts.

All you need to do is open a bottle 2 times per day, swallow it down and you're done.

Unfortunately though, not all multivitamin supplements are created equal. To understand this fully you need to understand the 2 standards of manufacturing that exist in the supplement industry today.

They are: Food grade and pharmaceutical grade.

Food grade products are made to the same standards food is made to. There's no guarantee that what's on the label is in the product and nor does there have to be. It's the same standard a food company will make a batch of cookies for example. There's no guarantee each cookie will have the same amount of chocolate chips and nor does their have to be.

Pharmaceutical grade products are made to the same strict standards employed by the pharmaceutical drug industry.

This means everything stated on the label is in the product every single time. There would be no contamination of ingredients such as pesticides and herbicides and heavy metals. And it's guaranteed to be broken down and absorbed by the body within 45 minutes.

You would assume all supplements are made to these standards but they're not. The supplement industry is largely unregulated meaning nobody is making sure companies are doing what they say they're doing.

Pharmaceutical grade manufacturing is totally voluntary and only a handful of companies in the world do it. We chose our product partner Usana Health Sciences based on the adoption of these pharmaceutical manufacturing standards. The company have also taken even more steps to set themselves apart from others in the industry.

Usana is the only nutritional company to manufacture their products in an FDA registered facility. They're achieved the highest product rating in the NutriSearch.ca **Comparative Guide to Nutritional Supplements.** (Link in the resources section)

In the latest edition, Nutrisearch had to create an entirely new category for Usana due to a recent upgrade to their products.

The upgrade included a patented combination of naturally occurring plant compounds called flavonoids. These compounds provide additional health benefits through cell-signaling, switching on your body's inherent antioxidant protection and renewal systems.

Flavonoids have also been shown to reduce the activity of a little known 'fat storage enzyme' called HSD - short for beta-hydroxysteroid dehydrogenase. HSD increases your fats cells sensitivity to cortisol which amplifies its fat storing effects.

Basically the HSD enzyme can reactivate inactive cortisol meaning your fat cells can produce their own fat storing cortisol even when stress levels are low.

Taking a high potency, pharmaceutical grade multivitamin also helps you prevent nutrient deficiency hunger cravings. Hunger cravings are the only way your body can communicate to you "give me nutrients" and it's the last thing you need when trying to stick to any meal plan.

If you crave the creaminess of ice cream, sour cream, milk, cheese and especially chocolate during menstruation, then calcium, magnesium and vitamin D are what your body needs. If you crave fatty and greasy foods it's usually a deficiency in fat soluble vitamins like vitamin E, D, K and essential fats. If you're having cravings for carbs like pastries and warm bread, then chances are you're low iodine.

Getting enough vitamins, minerals, antioxidants, phytonutrients and all the other micronutrients your body needs is crucial for your body to perform at its best and amplify your fat burning efforts.

If you develop this habit, using Usana Health Sciences multivitamin supplement, most people notice quite a dramatic change in their energy at first followed by an improvement in sleep, brighter eyes, skin and nails. Improved immunity, faster recovery from exercise and a feeling of increased wellbeing and vitality.

The multivitamin supplement I use and recommend is called **Cellsentials™** and **Prenatal CellSentials™** for pregnant women.

You can **buy Cellsentials™ and Prenatal CellSentials™ from my online store here.** (Link in the resources section)

The difference between the Prenatal CellSentials™ and Cellsentials™ is the prenatal includes iron and higher levels of iodine and folic acid.

Personally I use the Prenatal CellSentials™ even though I'm not pregnant. I'm low in iron so it saves me having to buy it elsewhere.

KEY LEARNINGS

- A multivitamin helps you prevent nutrient deficiency hunger cravings.
- Pharmaceutical grade products are made to the same strict standards employed by the pharmaceutical drug industry.
- Usana is the only nutritional company to manufacture their products in an FDA registered facility.
- The HSD enzyme can reactivate inactive cortisol meaning your fat cells can produce their own fat storing cortisol even when stress levels are low.
- Flavonoids contained in the Usana multivitamin have also been shown to reduce the activity of the 'fat storage enzyme' HSD.

HABIT #9
I have a modest exercise program. One that is aligned to my goals

Its no surprise that exercise is one of the 10 habits. You knew it was coming, but I bet you don't know why it's so important. Most people think the purpose of exercise is to burn fat. When in reality, the calories burned during exercise are very few.

The real purpose of exercise is to trigger fat burning hormones, so that post exercise, while you rest, your body can use those hormones to burn fat.

Most of your fat burning potential happens through the night when you are sleeping. Unless you are not sleeping very well but we'll deal with that in the next chapter.

The trick, is to stress the body just enough to stimulate fat burning hormones but not enough to produce fat storing hormones. The trouble is, the exercises that produce the most amount of fat burning hormones are the same exercises that trigger the most stress.

High Intensity exercises such as sprints, bodyweight exercises, lifting, jumping and bounding all create more stress and more fat burning hormones.

An unstressed (healthy) body, will very quickly adapt to the stress of high intensity exercise, which in turn increases its ability to handle more stress. However, if your body is already under stress, be it a physical, mental or even emotional stress, high intensity exercise is a no no.

Start with low intensity, aerobic exercise like walking, swimming, yoga, or cycling, and if you have a base of cardiovascular fitness then jogging, long distance cycling or running.

Your stress bucket has a limited capacity so a reduction in exercise intensity can keep cortisol low enough for long enough to start seeing results with exercise. You must align your exercise regime with your ability to manage the stress it creates. As that improves you can progress to higher and higher intensity.

I would like to share with you another reason why I think you absolutely must develop the habit of modest exercise in your life.

I refer to it as being 'ninja ready'. Its when someone calls and invites you to do something that involves moving your body (usually last minute) and you have the confidence in yourself to say yes. Its when you're open to experiencing something new.

Its when you can engage in all activities with your children, your nieces and nephews or grandchildren and connect with them on their terms. When you have the mobility and strength to squat down to their level.

Its when you drop something under your car and you get down horizontal to the ground in a plank position and can reach what you need.

Its when you're the one doing the inviting and planning fun activities and finally its when you get to feel the rush of pushing the limits of your body and breaking through to new levels.

Your body confidence is directly related to your ability to create a habit around exercise.

The best way to implement this habit is to simply start where you are and each week increase the following variables: frequency, the level of difficulty or intensity, the distance or duration. Do this in relation to the quality of sleep you are getting.

If you do not develop the habit of exercise in your life you will struggle with weight loss plateaus and you'll need to keep lowering your calories in order to lose weight.

Unfortunately as you lower your calories your thyroid will slow down its output and conversion of hormones crucial to the speed of your metabolism.

Initially this may not pose much of a problem but functioning on low calories can cause stress, inflammation and a drop in libido. The appetite controlling hormone called leptin, can slow down leaving you with wicked cravings.

You will lose weight but at what cost? It's extremely difficult to maintain and leads to yo-yo dieting and for someone caught in this cycle it means calories need to lowered more and more to lose weight.

On the flip side. If you push through the challenge of starting to regularly exercise and actually develop a habit in this area, your world will expand. Truly, confidence comes from feeling self assured in your body.

Exercise actually helps trigger growth hormones which are not only fat burning but are also anti-ageing as well. It also promotes muscle growth or muscle maintenance which improves your metabolism. Not to mention the long term benefits of improved cardiovascular health.

Your energy will improve and you may even become a morning person. You'll get ready quicker because you look good in your clothes. When you ask your partner "do I look good in this?" you'll believe him and you'll have better sex. You'll make new friends, have new experiences, and better holidays. You'll inspire people and become a role model whether you want to be or not. You'll eat better because when you prioritise exercise, you are showing yourself and the world that you are valuable.

KEY LEARNINGS

- The real purpose of exercise is to trigger fat burning hormones, so that post exercise, while you rest, your body can use those hormones to burn fat.
- The trick, is to stress the body just enough to stimulate fat burning hormones but not enough to produce fat storing hormones.
- Align your exercise regime with your ability to manage the stress it creates.
- Start where you are and each week increase the following variables: frequency, the level of difficulty or intensity, the distance or duration.
- Exercise helps trigger growth hormones which are fat burning and anti-ageing.

HABIT #10
I get adequate rest and recovery

Mastering this last habit is so important when it comes to fat loss. You already know **your body does most of its fat burning while you sleep** but let's be honest, most of us aren't getting quality of sleep needed to fully maximise this benefit.

To understand why we have trouble sleeping you need to know about a part of your nervous system called the autonomic nervous system. Your autonomic nervous system is responsible for controlling your bodily functions that are not consciously directed, such as breathing, your heartbeat, and your digestion.

Within the ANS you have 2 systems called the sympathetic and parasympathetic nervous systems. The parasympathetic nervous system serves to slow the heart rate and relax your muscles. This is the nervous system we need to be firing in order to get a great night's sleep.

Your sympathetic nervous system, on the other hand, activates the fight or flight response. This part of the ANS serves us very well when we need to get out of a potentially life threatening situation. But the problem is, the sympathetic nervous system can activate the fight or flight response even in times of perceived or imagined stress.

These are situations that are not an immediate threat to your safety. They're situations like the threat of losing your job, the instability of a relationship. Financial hardship, the fear of public speaking, work deadlines, even exercise. Basically everyday situations can trigger it. The problem with the sympathetic nervous system firing away all day long is that at some point you reach your limit. Stress does accumulate and you only have a limited capacity for it.

If you don't have strategies in place to deal with the accumulated stress, you'll be at your limit daily. When you're here your sleep is seriously impaired and your body will not be able to release fat naturally.

So bottom line, for our parasympathetic nervous system to be activated you must have strategies in place to release accumulated stress and empty our stress bucket.

Here are the best ways I've found to reduce stress and manage the balance of both the parasympathetic and sympathetic nervous system.

Eliminate highly caffeinated beverages including from diet drinks. Yip you did read that correctly. Gone. With the exception of coffee provided it's consumed with no milk and sugar. Alternatively use cream or coconut cream and stevia to sweeten. Provided you are able to maintain a low sugar and managed carbohydrate diet. Otherwise caffeine has a direct line of communication to your fight or flight nervous system.

Meditate. When you meditate, blood flow is increased to the part of the brain responsible for self-esteem, happiness, contentment, and peace.

Improving your diet by following the previous health habits mentioned in this book.

Getting the right ratio of high:low intensity exercise for your dominant hormonal weakness.

Supplementing with magnesium. Magnesium calms the sympathetic nervous activity helping your body to relax. You'll find balanced levels of magnesium in the **Cellsentials**™ multivitamin I mentioned in the previous chapter but in most cases additional magnesium is required to restore balance in this area. You can find additional magnesium in the **MagneCal D™** supplement I mentioned in chapter 7.

Supplementing with vitamin D. In some cases, therapeutic doses of 3000IU to 7000IU per day are needed to reduce stress and improve sleep. The Vitamin D supplement I use and recommend is from Usana Health Sciences.

You can **buy Vitamin D from my online store here.** (Link in the resources section)

Supplementing with B Vitamins. Especially B6 and B12 are important for calming the nervous system and mind. They also help with detoxification and lowering inflammation. You'll find optimal levels B vitamins in the Cellsentials™ multivitamin mentioned in the previous chapter.

Supplementing with Melatonin. This is very helpful for restoring sleep cycles.

Drinking chamomile tea. It has a mild sedative effect and may calm your brain and help you go to sleep sooner.

Dimming the interior lights of your home in the evening, taking a warm bath about 2 hours prior to bedtime, and no television or reading from a mobile phone prior to sleep.

If you don't get your nervous system operating in balance you'll experience... restless sleep, waking in the night to pee, having trouble getting back to sleep and racing mind. You'll wake in the morning feeling unrested. You'll have terrible workouts, slow recovery, poor energy and low libido.

Feeling the way I've just described is perfect grounds for overeating, and the associated guilt that goes along with it.

Anxiety is common place and overwhelming feelings of stress leading to panic attacks is quite possible. Also feelings of depression, becoming insular and spending less and less time with friends and family.

When you start to implement these things you'll feel a peace that only comes when you can sleep. Energy and vitality that comes when your body produces more serotonin, the happy hormone.

KEY LEARNINGS

- Your body does most of its fat burning while you sleep.
- The parasympathetic nervous system serves to slow the heart rate, relax your muscles and give you a great night's sleep.
- You must have strategies in place to release accumulated stress and empty your stress bucket.
- If you don't get your nervous system operating in balance you'll find it very difficult to lose weight.

Implementing the 10 Health Habits

Everyday you make decisions about what you eat and what you won't eat, how you'll move and relax, and with whom you spend time with.

Some of those decisions are conscious but most of them are being made in the subconscious part of your brain, they are what we call - your habits.

During times of pressure and stress we always default back to our subconscious behaviours aka our habits.

As you start to implement the 10 Health Habits from this book just be aware, a lot of the decisions you're making will come from the conscious part of your brain. They won't be real habits yet.

Some of the 10 Health Habits require practice and planning. A new way of shopping, eating and thinking. All of them require implementing. There's a lot going on, so when you experience feelings of overwhelm don't berate yourself if you slip back into you old ways.

That's completely normal. It doesn't mean you've failed, it just means that you're a human being who is habitually driven.

So watch the way you talk to yourself. Be patient with yourself and be kind.

I hope that I have given you enough compelling reasons to implement the 10 Health Habits you must to develop to finally free yourself from yo-yo dieting and start living in the body you've been wishing for.

Follow them and you will achieve your goals and develop a healthy lifestyle which has the side effect of permanent fat loss.

Are you ready to take it on? I'm assuming you are because you read all the way to the end of my book.

Nothing would give me more satisfaction than to support you in making that decision long term. It's not going to be an easy decision to keep making so I want to give you a fail safe plan to follow that I know will get you to your goal if you choose to keep following it.

Step 1 of the plan is take a quick and easy self evaluation. This self evaluation will rate your compliance with each of the 10 Health Habits. You'll get a score out of 50 which will serve as a starting point in your health habit journey. It doesn't matter what the score is, it's simply a starting point so be honest with yourself.

Step 2 of the plan is to identify 1-3 areas you can improve on and focus on them for the next month.

Step 3 is to take the self evaluation again and record your progress.

Step 4 is to repeat steps 2 & 3 until you've created all 10 Health Habits.

To begin the self evaluation process we're going to work through each Health Habit scoring yourself on a scale from 0-5 based on your level of compliance. I'll describe exactly what each level of compliance looks like so you can score yourself accurately.

Here's what the scores mean. 0= Don't know, 1= NOT, 2= A LITTLE, 3= SOMEWHAT, 4= MOSTLY, 5= FULLY!

So grab a pen and paper or open a notes app and let's begin:

How to do a Self Evaluation

Habit #1
I eat within 30 minutes of waking up and I do not eat within 2 hours of going to bed.

This habit is about starting and finishing your day well. Even if your day did not go as well as you had planned, you can still finish well.

• You will score yourself a 0 if you cannot remember whether you ate in the morning, or how late you ate before you went to bed.
• Score yourself a 1 if you skip breakfast and eat late into the evenings.
• Score yourself a 2 if you eat within 30 minutes of waking up and you do not eat within 2 hours of going to bed 3 days out of 7.
• Score yourself a 3 if you eat within 30 minutes of waking up and you do not eat within 2 hours of going to bed 4 days out of 7.
• Score yourself a 4 if you eat within 30 minutes of waking up and you do not eat within 2 hours of going to bed 5 days out of 7.
• Score yourself a 5 if you eat within 30 minutes of waking up and you do not eat within 2 hours of going to bed at least 6 days out of 7.

Habit 1 SCORE ___________

Habit #2
I eat every 3 hours. If I'm hungry before then I'll eat and adjust my time accordingly.

This habit is about meal preparation, meal timing listening to your body's cues.

• You will score yourself a 0 if you are unaware of the times you should be eating.
• Score yourself a 1 if you are aware of your eating times, but you're going too long between meals.

• Score yourself a 2 if you are aware of your eating times, listening to your hunger cues and managing your meals.
• Score yourself a 3 if you are aware of your hunger cues and you're managing your meals and snacks 3 days out of 7.
• Score yourself a 4 if you are aware of your hunger cues, and you're managing your meals and snacks 5 days out of 7.
• Score yourself a 5 if you are aware of your hunger cues, you can manage your meals and snacks 6 days out of 7 and adjust if them around your activity levels.

Habit 2 SCORE ___________

Habit #3
I eat according to my goals. Low GL to lose weight, and Medium GL to maintain.

This habit is about managing your carbohydrate intake so you don't spike your blood sugar.

• You will score yourself a 0 if you if you don't know what Glycemic Load means.
• Score yourself a 1 if you know what Glycemic Load means and you know what GL your meals and snack need to be to achieve your goal.
• Score yourself a 2 if you are eating low GL for 1 main meal per day.
• Score yourself a 3 if you are eating low GL for 2 main meals per day, 4 days out of 7.
• Score yourself a 4 if you are eating low GL for 3 main meals and 2 snacks per day, 5 days out of 7.
• Score yourself a 5 if you are eating low GL for 3 main meals and 2 snacks per day, 5 days out of 7. And you're able to adjust your GL depending on your activity level.

Habit 3 SCORE ___________

Habit #4
I eat enough protein with my meals and snacks.

This habit is about knowing how much and what kind of protein to consume for your body type and activity level.

- You will score yourself a 0 if you do not know how much protein you need and you don't know how much you're eating per day.
- Score yourself a 1 if you do know how much protein you need but you are not aware of how much you're eating per day.
- Score yourself a 2 if you know how much protein you need and you know how much you're eating per day.
- Score yourself a 3 if you know how much protein you need and you're achieving your daily protein goal 3 days out of 7.
- Score yourself a 4 if you know how much protein you need and you're achieving your daily protein goal 5 days out of 7.
- Score yourself a 5 if you know how much protein you need and you're achieving your daily protein goal 6 days out of 7. And you're able to adjust your protein intake according to your activity level.

Habit 4 SCORE ___________

Habit #5
I eat good fats with my meals and snacks. Especially the Omega 3's

This habit is about recognising the difference between different fats. Developing an optimal ratio of omega 3's and 6's, knowing how much fats you need to eat daily and taking a practitioner grade fish oil supplement.

- You will score yourself a 0 if you do not know the difference between omega 3, omega 6 and saturated fats.

- Score yourself a 1 if you know the difference between different fats but you are not considering your intake of omega 3's and 6's. Nor do you know how much fats you need daily.
- Score yourself a 2 if you know the difference between different fats, you've stopped cooking with vegetable oils, you know how much fats you need daily, and you're consuming omega 3's and 6's at least 3 x per week.
- Score yourself a 3 if you know the difference between different fats, you've stopped cooking with vegetable oils, you know how much fats you need daily, and you're consuming omega 3's and 6's at least 5 x per week.
- Score yourself a 4 if you know the difference between different fats, you've stopped cooking with vegetable oils, you know how much fats you need daily, and you're consuming omega 3's and 6's at least 5 x per week. You are also including a high quality pharmaceutical grade fish oil capsule 2x per day.
- Score yourself a 5 if you know the difference between different fats, you've stopped cooking with vegetable oils, you know how much fats you need daily, and you're consuming omega 3's and 6's at least 6 x per week. You are also taking a high quality pharmaceutical grade fish oil capsule 2x per day.

Habit 5 SCORE ___________

Habit #6
I get at least 35 grams of fibre per day.

This habit is about good gut health, and understanding that a healthy working bowel system is key to weight loss and excellent health. Knowing which foods contain high fibre and incorporating them along with a fibre supplement.

- You will score yourself a 0 if you do not know how much fibre you need per day
- Score yourself a 1 if you know how much fibre you need but you do not know how much fibre you are consuming per day.

• Score yourself a 2 if you know the highest fibre foods and you're consuming at least 20 grams per day 3 x per week.
• Score yourself a 3 if you know the highest fibre foods and you're consuming at least 20 grams per day 4 x per week.
• Score yourself a 4 if you know the highest fibre foods and you're consuming at least 35 grams per day with the help of a fibre supplement 3 x per week.
• Score yourself a 5 if you know the highest fibre foods and you're consuming at least 35 grams per day with the help of a fibre supplement 5 x per week.

Habit 6 SCORE ___________

Habit #7
I stay hydrated throughout the day.

This habit is about recognising that a focus on optimal vegetable intake is required for proper hydration.

• You will score yourself a 0 if you do not know the optimal servings of vegetable intake per day.
• Score yourself a 1 if you are consuming at least 2 servings per day at least 2 days per week.
• Score yourself a 2 if you are consuming at least 3 servings per day at least 3 days per week.
• Score yourself a 3 if you are consuming at least 5 servings per day at least 3 days per week.
• Score yourself a 4 if you are consuming 7 or more servings per day at least 4 days per week and the majority of those servings are dark leafy greens such as spinach, kale, silver beet.
• Score yourself a 5 if you are consuming 7 or more servings per day, 5 or more days per week and the majority of those servings are dark leafy greens such as spinach, kale, silver beet.

Habit 7 SCORE ___________

Habit #8
I take a high potency, pharmaceutical grade multivitamin 2X a day.

This habit is about understanding that optimal health needs optimal micro nutrition that can only be achieved when supplementing with a high potency, pharmaceutical grade multivitamin 2x per day.

- You will score yourself a 0 if you do not consume a pharmaceutical grade vitamin
- Score yourself a 1 if you consume your vitamins 1x per day, some days.
- Score yourself a 2 if you consume your vitamins 1x per day, most days.
- Score yourself a 3 if you consume your vitamins 2x per day, 4 days out of 7.
- Score yourself a 4 if you consume your vitamins 2x per day, 6 days out of 7
- Score yourself a 5 if you consume your vitamins 2x per day, 7 days out of 7.

Habit 8 SCORE ___________

Habit #9
I have a modest exercise program. One that is aligned to my goals.

This habit is about knowing the difference between high and low intensity exercise, aligning your exercise regime with your ability to manage the stress and starting where you are by increasing the following variables: frequency, the level of difficulty or intensity, the distance or duration.

- You will score yourself a 0 if you do not know the difference between high intensity and low intensity exercise.

• Score yourself a 1 if you know the difference between high intensity and low intensity exercise but you are practising neither for a focused period of time.
• Score yourself a 2 if you are exercising for any duration and any intensity, a minimum of 3 days per week
• Score yourself a 3 if you are exercising at least 30 mins 4x per week and you're progressing your intensity, duration, frequency or distance.
• Score yourself a 4 if you're doing both anaerobic and aerobic exercise at least 4x per week and you're progressing your intensity, duration, frequency or distance.
• Score yourself a 5 if you are practising both high and low intensity exercise at least 4x per week, you're progressing your intensity, duration, frequency or distance and you can lift or press your own body weight.

Habit 9 SCORE ___________

Habit #10
I get adequate rest and recovery

This habit is about understanding the true value of recovery. Not over exercising, and developing a good sleep routine so you can maximise your fat burning potential.

• You will score yourself a 0 if you do not know how to create an end of day routine.
• Score yourself a 1 if you do not have an end of day routine or you are not aerobically exercising.
• Score yourself a 2 if you are getting into deep sleep 3x per week, you have an end of day routine and you're exercising 2x per week.
• Score yourself a 3 if you are getting into deep sleep 4x per week, you have an end of day routine and you're exercising 3x per week.

• Score yourself a 4 if you are getting into deep sleep 5x per week, you have an end of day routine and you're exercising 4x per week. Also you're NOT doing high intensity exercise back to back.
• Score yourself a 5 if you are getting into deep sleep 5x per week, you have an end of day routine and you're exercising 4x per week or more. Also you're NOT doing high intensity exercise back to back, you're stretching at least 3x per week, you're practising meditation or diaphragmatic breathing.

Habit 10 SCORE ___________

MY TOTAL SCORE:___________ POSSIBLE SCORE: 50

Self Evaluation Form

LEVEL OF COMPLIANCE: 0= Don't know 1= NOT 2= A LITTLE 3= SOMEWHAT 4= MOSTLY 5= FULLY!

1. I eat within 30 minutes of waking up and I do not eat within 2 hours of going to bed.

    0   1   2   3   4   5

2. I eat every 3 hours. If I'm hungry before then I'll eat and adjust my time accordingly.

    0   1   2   3   4   5

3. I eat according to my goals. Low GL to lose weight, and Medium GL to maintain.

    0   1   2   3   4   5

4. I eat enough protein with my meals and snacks.

    0   1   2   3   4   5

5. I eat good fats with my meals and snacks. Especially Omega 3's

    0   1   2   3   4   5

6. I get at least 35 grams of fibre per day.

    0   1   2   3   4   5

7. I stay hydrated throughout the day.

    0   1   2   3   4   5

8. I take a high potency, pharmaceutical grade multivitamin 2X a day.

    0   1   2   3   4   5

9. I have a modest exercise program. One that is aligned to my goals.

    0   1   2   3   4   5

10. I get adequate rest and recovery

    0   1   2   3   4   5

MY TOTAL SCORE:__________ POSSIBLE SCORE: 50

Your BEST Next Move

I know how difficult it is to go on a weight loss journey alone, and I know a huge reason I was so successful in my journey is that I always had an awesome group of peers and mentors around me.

As a thank you for reading my book please join me in my **Be Free From Dieting** community Facebook group. (Link in the resources section)

Introduce yourself in the group and share with us your top takeaways from the book.

You can ask any question you have and myself or the other members of the group will answer it as soon as we can.

I provide free training, tips and motivation on weight loss, health and beauty but I created the group to support you on your journey so please make the most of it.

If you haven't already please like my **Facebook fan page** and leave a review of the book. It would would really help this message get out there.

If you're ready to take your health to the next level then your BEST Next Move is to take my online nutrition course called **GenHealth Coaching Program (GCP)**

The GenHealth Coaching Program is my proven, simple to follow system that works for virtually any person regardless of their age, weight or body type.

Unlike most courses, training and diet programs that only give you one piece of the puzzle – often times leaving you more confused, frustrated and overwhelmed than when you started (not to mention a few hundred or thousand bucks) – The GenHealth Coaching Program is the puzzle itself.

All you have to do is complete the right steps in the right order and we'll be right alongside you every step of the way!

Go to www.genhealthcoachingprogram.com for more information about my online program.

As you start implementing the 10 Health Habits please reach out to me and tell me how awesome you're feeling. Nothing will bring me more satisfaction than to hear your success stories. And better yet, share what you've learnt with those you care about the most.

To Your Weight Loss Success,

Tarryn Thompson
Your Virtual Health Coach
Creator of **GenHealth Coaching Program** & **Be Free From Dieting Formula**

FREE RESOURCES

Go to www.generationhealth.co.nz/resources for all the free resources mentioned in this book.

Go to www.generationhealthnz.usana.com for all Usana Foods and Vitamins mentioned in this book.

Go to www.generationhealth.co.nz.quiz for the Body Type Quiz mentioned in this book.